EZ LI...
A TO Z
CALORIE COUNTER©

By: Helena Schaar

ISBN # 1-4116-0282-X

Printed in the United States of America.
Published by Excel Services.
Send all correspondence to
excelservices222@yahoo.com.

This book is dedicated to my son, Jasen,
whom I love with all my heart and soul.

EZ LIFETIME
A TO Z
CALORIE COUNTER©

By: Helena Schaar

TABLE OF CONTENTS   ***Page No.***

- Introduction................................4
  - Tips on Using This Book
  - Abbreviation Key
  - Metric Conversion Factors
  - Measure Equivalents

- **Calorie Counters**
  - **Beverages...........................11**
  - **Foods..................................17**
  - **Fast Food Restaurants.............68**

- EZ! Lifetime Diet & Exercise Guide...77
  - Healthy Diet Basics
  - All About Calories & Weight
  - Calorie Expenditure & Exercise
  - EZ! Weight Loss Secrets
  - Ideal Body Weight Chart

- Free Access to Internet Site with
  Complete Food Nutritional Values.....98

*E-book online layout may have different page numbers depending on your browser.

INTRODUCTION

Welcome to the EZ Lifetime A to Z Calorie Counter©. You now possess the power to control your weight forever. This is a guide to safe, simple, effective methods of managing your weight, while promoting optimal health.

Nutrition experts agree, calories count first in weight management. This book is designed to help you count calories accurately, quickly, and easily. Alphabetical listings make locating your foods simple. To improve clarity and speed in locating food choices, this book is divided into 3 sections:

Beverages
Foods
Fast Food Restaurants

This edition is small and slim sized to easily fit into a purse or briefcase. Use it at home while planning meals and carry it wherever you go.

References for compiling this book are the United States Department of Agriculture (USDA) nutritional database, and food manufacturers' nutrient labels. References for the diet and exercise data are the USDA database and WebMD.com.

Counting calories is a time-honored method for weight management. Nutrition experts agree that <u>calories count first when trying to manage your weight.</u> Other factors can then be addressed, including your activity level, amount of daily exercise, and how you balance your intake of carbohydrates, protein, fat, sodium, and other nutrients.

This book is designed to help make counting calories fast and easy. Precise and accurate alphabetical listings provide for quick calorie counts. Whether you are a pro, or a novice at counting calories, you will find this book contains all the information you need for counting calories. Inside are all the foods you love to eat, prepared the ways most people love to eat them, in the most common serving sizes. This includes the most popular foods, the most common foods, favorite fast food restaurants, brand names, beverages, and alcoholic beverages.

Managing your weight is so much easier with the right tools, including a good calorie counter, and a simple exercise plan. This calorie counter includes the EZ! Lifetime Diet & Exercise Guide. Here, find all of the essential tools to manage your weight, and shed those unwanted pounds and inches forever. This book gives you the power base for building a lifetime of good health, and the joy of achieving your ideal body weight.

TIPS ON USING THIS BOOK

To use the calorie counter, simply locate your choice of food or beverage in one of the three alphabetical sections:

Beverages
Foods
Fast Food Restaurants

For the best results, read over the entire book to get an idea of which foods are high in calories and which foods are low in calories. That will help you make smart food choices every time you eat.

Also included in this book is the EZ! Lifetime Diet & Exercise Guide. This will give you all the information you need to understand calories, healthy dieting, and exercise. You can calculate your daily caloric requirements for achieving and maintaining your ideal weight. Calorie expenditure is also covered, including how to burn calories faster, exercise, and lifestyle activity levels. Also inside are plenty of diet tips and secrets. Calorie counting along with a simple exercise routine results in healthy weight management, with long-lasting results.

Whenever you need complete food nutritional values, turn to the section listing the free internet database with complete food counts. This includes carbohydrates, protein, fat, fiber, sodium, cholesterol counts and much more. This data can be downloaded to a computer, saved, and printed.

ABBREVIATION KEY:

appx	approximately
as prep	prepared as instructed on package, usual method
avg	average size
bev	beverage
dia	diameter
fl oz	fluid ounce
g	gram
"	inch(es)
Lb	pound
Lg	large
mcg	microgram
med	medium
misc	miscellaneous
mg	milligram
ml	milliliter
oz	ounce
pc	piece
pkg	package
pkt	packet
prep	prepared
sm	small
svg	serving
sq	square
Tbsp	tablespoon
Tr	trace- less than 1 g or mg
tsp	teaspoon
w/	with
w/o	without

Notes:

All listings are medium size or average portion size, unless specifically noted.

"Average calories" are used for foods with nearly identical calorie counts that are available from numerous food manufacturers. This keeps the book brief, without the unnecessary repetition and wordiness of multiple pages listing the same food. The calories listed represent an average of the compiled data

"Cooked" means the food is cooked without added fats, sauces, or sugars. This includes boiling and steaming.

"Baked" and "Broiled" mean the normal methods of baking and broiling, with minimal cooking oil for a non-stick surface. No other fats, sauces, or sugars added.

Italics signify registered trademarks for foods and restaurants.

The data is accurate at the time publication. However, food manufacturers may change their ingredients at any time without notice. Food nutrition labels should also be checked.

Metric Conversion Factors:

Volume	Multiply By	To Find Equivalent
Teaspoons	4.93	Milliliters
Tablespoons	14.79	Milliliters
Fluid ounces	29.57	Milliliters
Cups	0.24	Liters
Gallons	3.79	Liters

Weight	Multiply By	To Find Equivalent
Ounces	28.35	Grams
Pounds	0.45	Kilograms

Approximate Measure Equivalents:

VOLUME

1 Teaspoon = ……………………………….…5 ml
1 Tablespoon =…..3 Teaspoons =…………15 ml
2 Tablespoons =….1 fl oz = ………………30 ml
4 Tablespoons =….¼ Cup = …2 fl oz = …..59 ml
16 Tablespoons =…1 Cup = …8 fl oz =…..237 ml

1 Cup =………...½ Pint =…….8 fl oz = ….. 237 ml
2 Cups =………...1 Pint =…….16 fl oz = …..474 ml
2 Pints = ……...1 Quart =….32 fl oz = … 946 ml
1 Gallon = ……4 Quarts =..128 fl oz =   3.79 Liters

WEIGHT

1 Ounce = 28 grams
1 Pound = 454 grams

*This table lists approximate metric equivalents for easy reference.

EZ LIFETIME
A TO *Z*
CALORIE COUNTER©

BEVERAGES

BEVERAGES: (See Food and Fast Food Restaurants listed separately)	SERVING SIZE	CALORIES
Apple cider	6 fl oz	85
Apple juice	6 fl oz	85
Apple-cranberry juice	6 fl oz	115
Apple-grape juice	6 fl oz	100
Apricot nectar	6 fl oz	105
Beer		
regular	12 fl oz	150
light	12 fl oz	100
Bourbon		
80 proof	1 fl oz	65
100 proof	1 fl oz	85
Brandy		
regular 80 proof	1 fl oz	65
regular 100 proof	1 fl oz	85
sweetened, fruit flavored	1 fl oz	100
Cocoa/Chocolate Beverage or Hot Cocoa		
regular – as prep	6 fl oz	150
diet – as prep	6 fl oz	35
Coffee, unsweetened		
brewed	6 fl oz	2

BEVERAGES: (See Food and Fast Food Restaurants listed separately)	SERVING SIZE	CALORIES
espresso	4 fl oz	10
instant 1 tsp powder-prep	6 fl oz	2
(add 15 calories for each tsp of sugar added)		
Coke - see Soda	…	…
Cola - see Soda	…	…
Cranberry juice	8 fl oz	140
Cranberry juice cocktail sweetened	6 fl oz	110
Crystal Light, all flavors	8 fl oz	5
Daiquiri	4 fl oz	225
Diet Cola – also see Soda	12 fl oz	0
Diet or sugarfree *Kool-Aid* **or fruit drink**	8 fl oz	5
Diet Soda – also see Soda	12 fl oz	0
Eggnog, plain	1 cup	345
Fruit flavored drink bottled, canned, or prep from powder		
regular, sugar sweetened	8 fl oz	100
diet, aspartame sweetened	8 fl oz	5
Fruit punch	8 fl oz	110
Gin		
80 proof	1 fl oz	65
100 proof	1 fl oz	85
Grape juice	8 fl oz	100
Grapefruit juice fresh, unsweetened canned or frozen,	6 fl oz	70

BEVERAGES: (See Food and Fast Food Restaurants listed separately)	SERVING SIZE	CALORIES
unsweetened, as prep canned or frozen,	6 fl oz	70
sweetened, as prep	6 fl oz	95
Hot Cocoa – see Cocoa	...	...
Kool-Aid sugar sweetened	8 fl oz	100
sugarfree- sweetened with aspartame	8 fl oz	5
Lemon juice fresh, canned, or bottled	1 Tbsp	5
Lemonade sugar sweetened	8 fl oz	100
sugarfree- sweetened with aspartame	8 fl oz	5
Lime juice fresh, canned, or bottled	1 Tbsp	5
Limeade, sugar sweetened	8 fl oz	100
Liqueur, coffee or fruit flavored, 53 proof	1.5 fl oz	175
Milk whole (3.3% fat)	8 fl oz	150
reduced fat (2% fat)	8 fl oz	120
lowfat (1% fat)	8 fl oz	105
skim – nonfat milk	8 fl oz	85
buttermilk	8 fl oz	100
chocolate milk – whole	8 fl oz	210
chocolate milk – lowfat 2%	8 fl oz	180
chocolate milk- lowfat 1%	8 fl oz	160
condensed, sweetened, undiluted	4 fl oz	490

BEVERAGES: (See Food and Fast Food Restaurants listed separately)	SERVING SIZE	CALORIES
dried powdered milk, nonfat, instant- as prep	8 fl oz	80
evaporated, whole milk, undiluted	4 fl oz	170
evaporated, skim milk, undiluted	4 fl oz	100
malted milk, prep from powder chocolate flavor, w/ 2% milk	8 fl oz	170
natural flavor, w/ 2% milk	8 fl oz	180
milk shake, chocolate	8 fl oz	275
strawberry, or vanilla	8 fl oz	270
Orange juice, unsweetened, fresh, canned, or frozen, prep	6 fl oz	80
Orange-mixed fruit drink	6 fl oz	90
Orange-mixed fruit juice	6 fl oz	85
Orange-pineapple juice	6 fl oz	85
Pepsi – see Soda	…	…
Pina Colada	4.5 fl oz	260
Pineapple juice, unsweetened	6 fl oz	105
Prune juice	6 fl oz	135
Rum 80 proof	1 fl oz	65
100 proof	1 fl oz	85
Scotch 80 proof	1 fl oz	65
100 proof	1 fl oz	85

Shake
  thick milk shake, avg calories
    chocolate
	12 oz	410

strawberry	12 oz	400

BEVERAGES: (See Food and Fast Food Restaurants listed separately)	SERVING SIZE	CALORIES
vanilla	12 oz	400
Soda / Soft Drinks (Carbonated)		
club soda	12 fl oz	0
cherry cola	12 fl oz	150
cola type, *Coke, Pepsi*	12 fl oz	150
diet colas, sugarfree, sweetened with aspartame	12 fl oz	0
fruit flavored cola	12 fl oz	150
ginger ale	12 fl oz	125
grape	12 fl oz	150
lemon lime	12 fl oz	150
orange	12 fl oz	150
pepper type, *Dr Pepper*	12 fl oz	160
root beer	12 fl oz	150
Sprite, 7 Up	12 fl oz	150
Soft Drinks – see Soda	...	...
Sport drink	12 fl oz	75
Sugarfree beverage (Also see individual listings)		
Sugarfree soda	12 fl oz	0
Sugarfree fruit flavored drink	8 fl oz	5
Tea brewed, instant, hot and iced		
regular, unsweetened	8 fl oz	2
regular, sugar sweetened	8 fl oz	50
fruit flavored w/ sugar added	8 fl oz	110
diet, sweetened w/aspartame	8 fl oz	2
Tomato juice	6 fl oz	30
Vegetable juice cocktail	6 fl oz	35

BEVERAGES: (See Food and Fast Food Restaurants listed separately)	SERVING SIZE	CALORIES
Vodka		
80 proof	1 fl oz	65
100 proof	1 fl oz	85
Water	8 fl oz	0
Whiskey		
80 proof	1 fl oz	65
100 proof	1 fl oz	85
Wine		
dessert, dry	4 fl oz	150
dessert, sweet	4 fl oz	180
table, red	4 fl oz	85
table, white	4 fl oz	80
wine coolers	8 fl oz	120

EZ LIFETIME
A TO *Z*
CALORIE COUNTER©

FOOD

FOOD: (See Beverages & Fast Food Restaurants listed separately)	SERVING SIZE	CALORIES
Alfalfa sprouts, fresh	½ cup	5
***All-Bran* cereal**, 1 oz	½ cup	70
Allspice	1 tsp	5
Almonds, about 22	1 oz	165
Anchovy, canned in oil, drained	6	50
Angel-hair pasta, as prep	1 cup	210
Anise seed	1 tsp	7
Apple butter	1 Tbsp	30
Apple chips	1 oz	100
Apple pastry filling	1 Tbsp	40
Apple fresh, medium, 2 ¾" dia peeled, sliced	 1 ½ cup	 80 30
Applesauce sweetened unsweetened	 ½ cup ½ cup	 95 50
Apricot fresh, medium, 12 per pound canned, in juice canned, in heavy syrup dried, unsweetened,	 3 ½ cup ½ cup	 50 60 105

FOOD: (See Beverages & Fast Food Restaurants listed separately)	SERVING SIZE	CALORIES
halves, cooked	½ cup	105
Arrowroot	1 Tbsp	18
Artichoke, Globe or French		
fresh, medium size, cooked	1	60
canned or frozen, hearts	2 pieces	35
Jerusalem artichoke, sliced	½ cup	60
Asparagus		
fresh, medium size spears	4 spears	15
fresh, cut and cooked	½ cup	20
canned	½ cup	20
Avocado dip	1 Tbsp	30
Avocado, medium size, 8 oz	1	300
Bacon bits		
imitation	1 Tbsp	20
real	1 Tbsp	60
Bacon dip	1 Tbsp	30
Bacon, as prep		
American, 2.4 oz	3 slices	130
Canadian bacon, 2 oz	3 slices	70
Bagel, 3" dia unless noted		
plain	1	160
cheese	1	170
cinnamon raisin	1	170
egg	1	165
multigrain	1	150
onion	1	160
x-large, 5" dia, multigrain	1	310
(with 1 Tbsp regular cream		
cheese, add 50 calories;		
with 1 Tbsp light cream		

FOOD: (See Beverages & Fast Food Restaurants listed separately)	SERVING SIZE	CALORIES
cheese, add 25 calories)		
Bagel chips	1 oz	125
Baked beans, canned		
plain or vegetarian	½ cup	140
barbecue, honey, or brown sugar	½ cup	170
with pork and tomato sauce	½ cup	150
with pork and sweet sauce	½ cup	170
Baking powder	1 Tbsp	10
Baking soda	1 Tbsp	1
Banana bread, ½" slice	1 slice	180
Banana split, avg	1	510
Banana, medium size	1	105
Barbecue sauce		
regular	1 Tbsp	25
extra thick, or honey flavor	1 Tbsp	40
Barley		
pearled, cooked	½ cup	95
Basil		
fresh, chopped	¼ cup	5
dried, ground	1 Tbsp	10
Bass		
freshwater, baked or broiled	3 oz	125
sea bass, baked or broiled	3 oz	105
Bean dip	1 Tbsp	20
Bean salad		
w/sweet and sour dressing	½ cup	70
Bean sprouts		
fresh, raw	½ cup	15
cooked	½ cup	30

FOOD: (See Beverages & Fast Food Restaurants listed separately)	SERVING SIZE	CALORIES
Bean with bacon soup	1 cup	170
Beans (also see mixed bean dishes listed individually)		
baked beans, plain, as prep	½ cup	140
green beans, fresh, raw	½ cup	18
green beans, fresh, cooked	½ cup	25
kidney/red beans, cooked	½ cup	110
lima beans, cooked	½ cup	100
pinto beans, cooked	½ cup	95
snap beans, green, cooked	½ cup	25
snap beans, yellow, cooked	½ cup	25
soybeans, dried mature seeds, cooked	½ cup	115
wax beans, cooked	½ cup	25
white beans, cooked	½ cup	120
Beef (weights for meat without bones)		
corned beef, canned	3 oz	210
chuck, lean stewing cut, braised	4 oz	245
flank steak, lean, braised	4 oz	230
ground beef, broiled (also see hamburger & cheeseburger)		
regular ground beef	3 oz	245
lean ground beef	3 oz	230
extra lean ground beef	3 oz	205
liver, fried	3 oz	275
lunch meat, thin sliced		
regular	2 slices	180
lowfat	2 slices	110
fat free	2 slices	60

FOOD: (See Beverages & Fast Food Restaurants listed separately)	SERVING SIZE	CALORIES
pot roast, braised or simmered	3 oz	200
porterhouse steak, lean, broiled	4 oz	255
ribs, roasted, lean and fat	3 oz	320
roast beef,		
regular roast beef	3 oz	220
lean roast beef	3 oz	160
sirloin steak, broiled,		
lean and fat	3 oz	240
lean only	3 oz	180
T-bone steak, broiled,		
lean and fat	4 oz	340
lean only	4 oz	250
tenderloin or top loin, broiled,		
lean and fat	4 oz	340
lean only	4 oz	250
Beef and vegetable stew	1 cup	175
Beef bouillon		
broth or consommé	1 cup	15
Beef noodle soup	1 cup	85
Beet greens, chopped, cooked	½ cup	20
Beets, sliced, cooked	½ cup	25
Black beans, canned	½ cup	100
Blackberries fresh or frozen	½ cup	50
Black-eyed peas	½ cup	100
Blintzes, misc variety, avg	1	100
Blue cheese, crumbled	¼ cup	120
Blueberries		
fresh	½ cup	40
canned or frozen, sweetened	½ cup	95
Bluefish, baked or broiled	3 oz	135

FOOD: (See Beverages & Fast Food Restaurants listed separately)	SERVING SIZE	CALORIES
Bok-choy cabbage, raw, shredded	1 cup	10
Bologna (calories are for the usual thin 1/8" slices; for thick ¼" slices, double the calories)		
fat free beef or pork	2 slices	60
fat free chicken or turkey	2 slices	50
low fat beef or pork	2 slices	110
low fat chicken or turkey	2 slices	100
regular beef or pork	2 slices	180
regular chicken or turkey	2 slices	160
Boston Cream Pie 1/12 of 8" pie	1 piece	225
Bouillon cubes beef, pork, or chicken 1 cup of prepared broth	1 cube	15
Bran flakes cereal, 1 oz	¾ cup	90
Braunschweiger	2 oz	205
Bread crumbs	¼ cup	100
Bread sticks, snack type, thin	6 pieces	70
Bread (also see individual listings) bagel, 3" dia unless noted		
plain	1	160
cheese	1	170
cinnamon raisin	1	170
egg	1	165
multigrain	1	150
onion	1	160
x-large, 5" dia, multigrain	1	310
banana bread, 1" slice	1 slice	165

FOOD: (See Beverages & Fast Food Restaurants listed separately)	SERVING SIZE	CALORIES
biscuit, avg 2 ½" dia	1 piece	120
bun, frankfurter, 1.4 oz, 5 ½"	1 piece	100
bun, hamburger, 1.4 oz 3 ½" dia	1 piece	100
cornbread 2 ½" dia	1 piece	110
croissant, plain, 4"	1 piece	150
English muffin, plain	1 piece	120
French bread, avg 1.4 oz slice	1 slice	110
hard roll, avg 1.2 oz	1 roll	85
Italian bread, avg 1.4 oz slice	1 slice	110
light bread, avg of all varieties	1 slice	45
oat/ oat bran bread, avg slice	1 slice	105
onion bread, avg slice	1 slice	80
pita bread 5 ¼" dia	1 pocket	130
potato bread, avg slice	1 slice	95
pumpernickel bread, avg 1 oz slice	1 slice	70
raisin bread, thin sliced	1 slice	70
roll (dinner) avg 1 oz, 2 ½" dia (also see rolls)	1 roll	75
rye bread, avg 0.9 oz slice	1 slice	70
sourdough bread, avg 0.8 oz slice	1 slice	65
submarine bun, 7" long, 2.8 oz bun	1 bun	190
thin sliced white/wheat bread	1 slice	55
Vienna bread, avg 1.4 oz slice	1 slice	110
white bread, avg 0.8 oz slice	1 slice	60
wheat bread, avg 0.8 oz slice	1 slice	60
Breakfast sandwich, with bacon, egg, and cheese		

FOOD: (See Beverages & Fast Food Restaurants listed separately)	SERVING SIZE	CALORIES
on English muffin	1 avg	385
Broccoli fresh, flowerets	3	10
fresh, spears and cuts, chopped, cooked	½ cup	22
frozen, spears and cuts, cooked	½ cup	28
broccoli in butter sauce	¾ cup	58
broccoli in cheese sauce	¾ cup	72
Brown sugar	1 tsp	15
	1 cup	720
Brownie, with nuts, 2" square		
with frosting	1 square	175
without frosting	1 square	130
Brussels sprouts, cooked	4 sprouts	35
Bulgur, cooked	1 cup	150
Bun, avg hamburger or hot dog	1	100
Burrito bean and cheese	1 avg	320
beef and bean	1 avg	390
Butter (also see margarine and individual listings) regular and stick	1 Tbsp	100
whipped	1 Tbsp	70
Butterfish, baked or broiled	3 oz	160
Butternuts, dried, shelled	1 oz	175
Butterscotch hard candy, 1" dia	1 piece	20
Butterscotch morsel for baking	1 oz	145
Butterscotch syrup regular	1 Tbsp	60
light/low calorie	1 Tbsp	25

FOOD: (See Beverages & Fast Food Restaurants listed separately)	SERVING SIZE	CALORIES
Cabbage,		
green, red, or savoy		
fresh, raw, sliced or shredded	1 cup	20
shredded, cooked	½ cup	15
bok-choy cabbage		
raw, shredded	1 cup	10
Cake (all cake listings are for an average size slice; all are 1 layer cakes unless noted)		
angelfood cake, w/o frosting	1 piece	145
banana cake, w/glaze	1 piece	250
carrot cake w/cream cheese		
frosting	1 piece	340
cheesecake	1 piece	410
chocolate cake w/frosting		
1 layer cake	1 piece	290
2 layer cake	1 piece	495
coffee crumb cake	1 piece	250
cupcake – see cupcake		
devils-food cake w/frosting		
1 layer cake	1 piece	290
2 layer cake	1 piece	495
fat free cake,		
chocolate, vanilla, or variety,		
w/o frosting	1 piece	150
w/sugar free frosting/glaze	1 piece	180
frosting for cake,		
regular	1 Tbsp	75
sugarfree	1 Tbsp	30

FOOD: (See Beverages & Fast Food Restaurants listed separately)	SERVING SIZE	CALORIES
fruitcake, dark	1 piece	330
gingerbread	1 piece	240
marble cake, w/o frosting	1 piece	240
pound cake, w/o frosting	1 piece	220
sponge cake, w/o frosting	1 piece	150
yellow cake		
w/o frosting 1 layer	1 piece	220
w/frosting, 2 layer	1 piece	475
Candy		
3 Musketeers, 2.1 oz bar	1 bar	260
Baby Ruth, 2.1 oz bar	1 bar	280
Butterfinger, 2.1 oz bar	1 bar	280
candy cane, 0.5 oz	1 piece	55
candy corn	10 pieces	35
caramels, 3 pieces/oz		
chocolate caramel	1 oz	85
plain caramel	1 oz	110
chocolate,		
Hershey's Kiss	2	50
Hershey's Nugget	1	50
milk chocolate bar, 1 ½ oz		
plain chocolate bar	1 bar	220
with almonds	1 bar	230
with crispy rice	1 bar	230
with nuts (1 ¾ oz bar)	1 bar	280
semisweet chocolate chips	¼ cup	215
chocolate covered raisins	1.5 oz	190
fruit bar	1 oz	80
gum, chewing		
regular gum, 3" stick	1 stick	10

FOOD: (See Beverages & Fast Food Restaurants listed separately)	SERVING SIZE	CALORIES
sugarfree gum, 3" stick	1 stick	5
Dentyne gum, 1 ¼" stick	1 stick	5
gum drops, 8 pieces/oz	1 oz	95
large gumball, 1 ¼"dia	1	30
hard candy, butterscotch, cinnamon, or fruit flavored	1 oz	105
1 piece, 1" dia	1 piece	20
hard candy, sugar free, *Sweet'N Low*, creme variety	1 piece	10
Sweet'N Low, misc varieties, except creme	1 piece	6
jelly beans, 10 pieces	1 oz	95
licorice, bite size	¼ cup	170
stick, 6 ½" long	1 stick	40
Shoestring, 43" long	1 piece	70
LifeSavers	1 piece	10
M&M candy-coated, plain	10 pieces	35
with peanut butter	10 pieces	35
with nuts	10 pieces	90
mints, pastel, ½" square	10 pieces	75
marshmallows, 4 pc, 1 1/8" dia	1 oz	90
Snickers, 2.1 oz bar	1 bar	280
Toffee, 1.5 oz	6 pieces	170
Tootsie roll, 1 ¼ oz roll	1 roll	140
Cantaloupe fresh, medium size melon	½ melon	120
fresh, cubed	1 cup	50
Caramels – see candy	…	…
Caraway seed	1 tsp	7

FOOD: (See Beverages & Fast Food Restaurants listed separately)	SERVING SIZE	CALORIES
Carp, meat only, broiled	3 oz	140
Carrots		
fresh, raw 7" x 1 ¾"	1	25
fresh, raw, shredded	½ cup	25
cooked, sliced	½ cup	35
Cashews, roasted, about 18	1 oz	160
Catfish		
baked or broiled	3 oz	105
fried	3 oz	180
Catsup	1 Tbsp	20
Cauliflower		
fresh flowerets, raw	4 pieces	10
fresh cuts and pieces, cooked	¾ cup	25
frozen cuts and pieces, cooked	¾ cup	30
Caviar, black or red, granular	1 oz	70
Celery		
fresh stalk 7 ½" x 1 ¼"	1 stalk	5
cooked, diced	½ cup	10
Cereal – see individual listings	…	…
Cereal bar, all types, avg	1 bar	130
Cheddar cheese – see cheese	…	…
Cheerios cereal, 1 oz	1 cup	110
Cheese		
American cheese, processed		
fat free, 0.7 ounce slice	1 slice	25
regular, 1 ounce slice	1 slice	100
1 inch cube	1 cube	65
shredded, 2 oz	½ cup	210
cheese food spread	1 Tbsp	50
blue cheese, crumbled	¼ cup	120

FOOD: (See Beverages & Fast Food Restaurants listed separately)	SERVING SIZE	CALORIES
cheddar cheese		
fat free, 0.7 ounce slice	1 slice	30
regular, 1 ounce slice	1 slice	115
1 inch cube	1 cube	70
shredded	½ cup	225
cheese food spread	1 Tbsp	50
Colby or Monterey Jack	1 oz	115
cottage cheese		
regular, creamed, 4% fat	½ cup	110
lowfat, 2% fat	½ cup	100
fat free	½ cup	80
cream cheese, regular	1 Tbsp	50
lowfat/light cream cheese	1 Tbsp	25
feta cheese, crumbled	¼ cup	90
mozzarella cheese		
fat free, 0.7 ounce slice	1 slice	20
regular, 1 ounce slice	1 slice	80
1 inch cube	1 cube	50
shredded, 2 oz	½ cup	170
muenster cheese		
sliced	1 oz	105
1 inch cube	1 cube	65
parmesan cheese	1 Tbsp	25
provolone cheese		
sliced	1 oz	100
1 inch cube	1 cube	60
ricotta cheese		
regular	¼ cup	110
fat free	¼ cup	60

FOOD: (See Beverages & Fast Food Restaurants listed separately)	SERVING SIZE	CALORIES
Swiss cheese		
fat free, 0.7 ounce slice	1 slice	25
regular, 1 ounce slice	1 slice	100
1 inch cube	1 cube	60
shredded, 2 oz	½ cup	200
Cheese puffs	10 pieces	85
snack size pkg, 2 oz	1 pkg	320
Cheeseburger		
with catsup, mustard, lettuce, tomato, and pickles		
2 oz patty	1 avg	340
4 oz patty	1 avg	530
Cherry		
fresh	½ cup	45
canned, sweet in juice	½ cup	70
canned, sweet in heavy syrup	½ cup	105
Chestnut, roasted, peeled	½ cup	175
Chewing gum – see gum	...	...
Chicken		
broiled, light & dark meat, without skin	3 oz	135
chicken liver, simmered	3 oz	160
fried, meat and skin	3 oz	230
fried, meat only	3 oz	175
fried, breaded, breast, meat & skin	½ breast	200
fried, breaded, drumstick, meat & skin	1 piece	130
fried, breaded, thigh, meat and skin	1 thigh	175

FOOD: (See Beverages & Fast Food Restaurants listed separately)	SERVING SIZE	CALORIES
fried, breaded, wing, meat and skin	1 wing	95
lunch meat, thin sliced		
regular	2 slices	160
lowfat	2 slices	100
fat free	2 slices	50
roasted chicken		
light meat without skin	3 oz	145
light meat with skin	3 oz	175
dark meat without skin	3 oz	155
dark meat with skin	3 oz	180
Chicken broth		
prep from bouillon cube	1 cup	15
Chicken noodle soup	1 cup	75
Chicken roll, light meat	3 oz	135
Chicken with rice soup	1 cup	75
Chickpeas, cooked	½ cup	150
Chili powder	1 tsp	8
Chili with beans	1 cup	305
Chips – see corn chips, potato chips & other individual listings	…	…
Chives, fresh, chopped	2 Tbsp	1
Chocolate (also see candy) milk chocolate bar, 1 ½ oz		
plain chocolate bar	1 bar	245
with almonds	1 bar	235
with crispy rice	1 bar	215
with peanuts (1 ¾ oz bar)	1 bar	280
M&M candy-coated, plain	10 pieces	35
with peanut butter	10 pieces	35

FOOD: (See Beverages & Fast Food Restaurants listed separately)	SERVING SIZE	CALORIES
with nuts	10 pieces	90
semisweet chocolate chips	¼ cup	215
Chocolate syrup		
regular	1 Tbsp	60
light/low calorie	1 Tbsp	25
Clam chowder		
Manhattan style	1 cup	80
New England style		
prep with water	1 cup	95
prep with milk	1 cup	145
Clams		
canned, in liquid	3 oz	80
fresh, hard or round, meat only	4 oz	80
fresh, soft, meat only	4 oz	95
Cloves, ground	1 tsp	7
Cocoa, for baking	1 Tbsp	15
Coconut		
fresh, grated	½ cup	140
dried, sweetened, flaked	2 Tbsp	45
Cod		
fresh, raw	3 oz	70
baked or broiled	3 oz	90
battered, fried	3 oz	170
Coffee cake, 2 ½" x 2"	1 piece	115
Colby cheese – see cheese	…	…
Coleslaw	½ cup	70
Collards, fresh, chopped, cooked	½ cup	10
Cookie, 2 ½" dia unless noted		
chocolate chip cookie	1	70
fig bar, 1 ½" square	1	55

FOOD: (See Beverages & Fast Food Restaurants listed separately)	SERVING SIZE	CALORIES
oatmeal cookie	1	60
oatmeal cookie w/raisins	1	65
peanut butter cookie	1	75
sandwich cookie, 1 ½" dia, chocolate or vanilla	1	55
shortbread cookie	1	70
sugar cookie	1	70
vanilla wafer, 1 ½" dia	2	40
Coriander, dried	1 tsp	4
Corn		
fresh, on cob 5" long	1	80
canned, kernels	½ cup	80
canned, cream style kernels	½ cup	90
Corn Chex **cereal**	1 ¼ cup	110
Corn chips		
regular size chips	10 chips	95
snack size pkg, 2 oz	1 pkg	310
barbecue, snack size pkg, 2 oz	1 pkg	320
king size chips	10 chips	150
Corn flakes cereal, 1 oz	1 cup	110
Corn grits (hominy), as prep	¾ cup	100
Corn Pops **cereal**, 1 oz	1 cup	105
Cornbread 2 ½" x 2"	1 piece	150
Corned beef hash	1 cup	395
Corned beef, canned	3 oz	210
Cornish hen, roasted	3 oz	190
Cornmeal	¼ cup	120
Cornstarch	1 Tbsp	30
Cottage cheese – see cheese	…	…

FOOD: (See Beverages & Fast Food Restaurants listed separately)	SERVING SIZE	CALORIES
Crab		
fresh, steamed, meat only	4 oz	110
canned	3 oz	80
imitation crabmeat	4 oz	120
Crackers		
butter flavor, round, 2" dia	5	80
cheese flavor, 1" squares	20	100
graham, 2 ½" squares	4	120
matzo, 6" square	1	120
oyster crackers	20	90
Ritz crackers, 2" dia	5	80
saltine crackers	8	100
sandwich crackers, 1 ½" dia,		
cheese filled	4	140
peanut butter filled	4	140
snack type, round, 2" dia	6	90
vegetable	6	75
wheat crackers 1 ¾" dia	6	90
Cranberry sauce	¼ cup	105
Cream cheese		
regular	1 Tbsp	50
lowfat/light	1 Tbsp	25
Cream of broccoli soup	1 cup	235
Cream of chicken soup		
prepared with water	1 cup	115
prepared with milk	1 cup	185
Cream of mushroom soup		
prepared with water	1 cup	130
prepared with milk	1 cup	190
Cream of wheat cereal	¾ cup	100

FOOD: (See Beverages & Fast Food Restaurants listed separately)	SERVING SIZE	CALORIES
Creamer		
liquid	1 Tbsp	20
powdered	1 Tbsp	10
sugar sweetened flavors	1 Tbsp	40
Croissant, plain, 4"	1	150
Cucumbers, fresh, unpeeled		
whole cucumber, med, 8" long	1	35
sliced cucumber	10 slices	12
Cumin seed	1 tsp	8
Cupcake, with frosting, 2 ¾" dia		
chocolate	1	160
vanilla	1	150
other varieties	1	155
Curry powder	1 tsp	6
Custard, baked	½ cup	130
Danish pastry, 4" dia	1	395
Dates, whole, pitted, dried	5	115
Dessert filling - see pastry filling	...	...
Dessert topping		
butterscotch or caramel, regular	1 Tbsp	60
light/low calorie	1 Tbsp	25
chocolate or fudge, regular	1 Tbsp	60
light/low calorie	1 Tbsp	25
fruit flavored, Regular	1 Tbsp	55
light/low calorie	1 Tbsp	20
whipped, white, frozen	2 Tbsp	30
whipped, white, pressurized	2 Tbsp	25
Doughnut, round, 3" dia		
cake type, plain	1	160
cake type, frosted	1	200

FOOD: (See Beverages & Fast Food Restaurants listed separately)	SERVING SIZE	CALORIES
cake type, filled and frosted	1	240
yeast type, glazed	1	220
yeast type, frosted	1	250
yeast type, filled and frosted	1	290
Dressing – see salad dressing	…	…
Dumpling, fruit flavor, avg	1	290
Éclair, chocolate, 2.1 oz piece	1 piece	150
Eel, meat only, baked or broiled	3 oz	190
Egg roll, with meat, 4"x 1 ½"	1	170
Egg substitute, or imitation	¼ cup	25
Eggs		
deviled	1 large	125
fried	1 large	95
hard or soft cooked	1 large	80
omelet, plain, milk added	1 large	105
poached	1 large	80
scrambled, milk added	1 large	105
Eggplant		
fresh, untrimmed	1 Lb	96
cubed, cooked	½ cup	15
cut, fried	½ cup	105
Elderberries, fresh	1 cup	100
Enchilada with beef & cheese	1 avg	325
Endive, raw, chopped	1 cup	7
English muffin, plain	1	130
Equal sweetener	1 pkt	0
Fajita, chicken, avg serving	1	460
Fennel, fresh, trimmed, sliced	¼ cup	15
Feta cheese – see cheese	…	…

FOOD: (See Beverages & Fast Food Restaurants listed separately)	SERVING SIZE	CALORIES
Fettuccine Alfredo, 8 oz serving	1	380
Fig bar, 1 ½" square	1	55
Fig, fresh, 1 large	1	45
Filling - see pastry filling	...	...
Fish, meat only, avg calories for white meat fish (also see specific individual listings)		
fresh, raw	3 oz	75
baked or broiled	3 oz	95
battered, fried	3 oz	175
Fish sandwich, 2 oz fried fish fillet		
with tarter sauce	1 avg	445
with tarter sauce & cheese	1 avg	525
Fish sticks, frozen, heated	3 pieces	150
Flank steak – see beef	...	...
Flatfish – see sole	...	...
Flounder		
fresh, raw	3 oz	80
baked or broiled	3 oz	100
battered, fried	3 oz	180
Flour		
oat flour	1 cup	480
rye flour, light or medium	1 cup	380
rye flour, whole grain	1 cup	640
white flour	1 cup	400
whole wheat flour	1 cup	400
Frankfurter (hot dog)		
beef or pork	1	140
chicken or turkey	1	115

FOOD: (See Beverages & Fast Food Restaurants listed separately)	SERVING SIZE	CALORIES
lowfat/light variety	1	75
fat free variety	1	45
French fries (fried potatoes)		
thin 3" strips	10	150
thick or crinkle cuts, 3" strips	10	195
French toast, avg calories	2 pieces	250
Fried chicken – see chicken	…	…
Fried rice, meatless	1 cup	270
with meat or seafood	1 cup	310
Frosted flakes, corn cereal, 1 oz	¾ cup	110
Frosted wheat cereal, 1 oz	½ cup	100
Frosting for cake, avg calories,		
regular	1 Tbsp	75
sugarfree	1 Tbsp	30
Frozen fruit juice bar	2 ½ fl oz	70
Fruit (see individual listings)		
mixed, canned, in light syrup	½ cup	80
Fruit cocktail, canned		
in heavy syrup	½ cup	90
in juice	½ cup	55
Fudge, chocolate or vanilla		
plain	1 oz	110
with nuts	1 oz	120
Garbanzos, cooked	½ cup	150
Garlic		
fresh	1 clove	4
powder	1 tsp	12
salt	1 tsp	3
Gelatin dessert, fruit flavored		
regular	½ cup	70

FOOD: (See Beverages & Fast Food Restaurants listed separately)	SERVING SIZE	CALORIES
sugarfree	½ cup	10
Gelatin, unflavored	1 pkg	25
Ginger		
trimmed root	1 oz	20
dried, ground	1 tsp	6
Goat, meat only, roasted	3 oz	120
Goose, roasted		
meat w/o skin	3 oz	200
meat with skin	3 oz	260
Gooseberry, fresh	½ cup	35
Granola bar		
low fat, misc varieties	1 bar	90
oats and chocolate chips	1 bar	150
oats and peanuts	1 bar	160
oats and raisins or coconut	1 bar	140
Granola cereal, 1 oz	¼ cup	130
Grapefruit, pink, red, or white		
fresh, med, 3 ¾" dia	1	80
canned, in juice	½ cup	45
canned, in light syrup	½ cup	75
Grape-Nut flakes cereal, 1 oz	¾ cup	100
Grapes, fresh,		
European, seeded	½ cup	57
seedless, med size	10 grapes	35
seedless, canned in water	½ cup	46
seedless, canned in heavy syrup	½ cup	95
Gravy		
beef or pork	2 Tbsp	30
chicken or turkey	2 Tbsp	25
mushroom	2 Tbsp	20

FOOD: (See Beverages & Fast Food Restaurants listed separately)	SERVING SIZE	CALORIES
Grits, corn, as prep	¾ cup	100
Ground beef – see beef	…	…
Grouper, baked or broiled	3 oz	100
Guava, medium size	1	45
Gum, chewing		
regular gum, 2 7/8" stick	1 stick	10
sugarfree gum, 2 7/8" stick	1 stick	5
Dentyne gum, 1 ¼" stick	1 stick	5
gum drops, 8 pieces/oz	1 oz	95
large gumball, 1 ¼"dia	1	30
Haddock		
fresh, raw	3 oz	75
baked or broiled	3 oz	95
battered, fried	3 oz	175
Half and half **cream**	1 Tbsp	20
Halibut, Atlantic or Pacific		
baked or broiled	3 oz	110
Ham, boneless (also see pork)		
canned, lean	3 oz	140
cured, roasted,		
lean and fat	3 oz	210
lean only	3 oz	130
fresh, baked		
lean and fat	3 oz	220
lean only	3 oz	140
lunch meat		
regular, avg calories	1 slice	75
lean, avg calories	1 slice	35
Hamburger (also see Ground Beef)		

FOOD: (See Beverages & Fast Food Restaurants listed separately)	SERVING SIZE	CALORIES
hamburger w/ catsup, mustard, lettuce, tomato, & pickles		
2 oz patty	1 avg	260
4 oz patty	1 avg	450
with 1 slice cheese, add 90 calories		
Hash browned potatoes	½ cup	175
Herring		
Atlantic, baked or broiled	3 oz	170
Pacific, baked or broiled	3 oz	210
Hominy grits, as prep	¾ cup	100
Honey	1 Tbsp	60
Honey Smacks cereal, 1 oz	¾ cup	105
Honeydew melon, fresh		
avg 6 ½" melon	¼ melon	110
avg 6 ½" melon, cubed	½ cup	30
Horseradish	1 Tbsp	5
Hot Dog – see frankfurter	…	…
Ice cream		
chocolate, vanilla, or strawberry		
lowfat	½ cup	90
regular, 10% fat	½ cup	135
rich, 16% fat	½ cup	175
ice cream bar, vanilla sandwich	1	220
ice cream cone, plain, unfilled	1	25
Jalapeno, whole, red	1 oz	15
Jams and Preserves,		
various flavors, regular	1 Tbsp	55
various flavors, light	1 Tbsp	25
Jellies, various fruit flavors	1 Tbsp	50

FOOD: (See Beverages & Fast Food Restaurants listed separately)	SERVING SIZE	CALORIES
Jello, gelatin, fruit flavored		
regular	½ cup	70
sugarfree	½ cup	10
Kale		
fresh, raw	½ cup	17
chopped, cooked	½ cup	22
Ketchup	1 Tbsp	20
Kiwifruit, fresh, medium size	1	45
Kumquat, fresh, medium size	1	12
Lamb		
ground lamb, broiled	3 oz	305
leg, roasted		
lean and fat	3 oz	235
lean only	3 oz	160
shoulder chop, broiled		
lean and fat	3 oz	285
lean only	3 oz	175
Lard	1 Tbsp	120
Lasagna, 2 ½" x 4 "	1 piece	330
Leek, fresh, chopped, cooked	½ cup	30
Lemon, fresh, 2 ¼" dia	1	25
Lentil, cooked	½ cup	115
Lettuce, fresh		
head of lettuce (iceberg), 6" dia	1 head	60
head of lettuce (Bibb, Boston), 5"dia	1 head	24
loose leaf, salad pieces	1 cup	5
wedge slice, iceberg, ¼ of 7"	1 wedge	10
Lime, fresh, 2" dia	1	20

FOOD: (See Beverages & Fast Food Restaurants listed separately)	SERVING SIZE	CALORIES
Liver		
beef liver, fried	3 oz	200
chicken liver, simmered	3 oz	160
turkey liver, simmered	3 oz	180
Lobster, meat only, steamed	4 oz	110
Lunch meat, (calories are for the usual thin 1/8" slices; for thick ¼" slices, double the calories)		
fat free beef or pork	2 slices	60
fat free chicken or turkey	2 slices	50
low fat beef or pork	2 slices	110
low fat chicken or turkey	2 slices	100
regular beef or pork	2 slices	180
regular chicken or turkey	2 slices	160
Lychee, raw, peeled	1 oz	18
Macadamia nut, dried, shelled	1 oz	200
Macaroni and cheese	1 cup	400
Macaroni, plain, cooked	1 cup	190
Mackerel, meat only		
Atlantic, baked or broiled	3 oz	220
Pacific, baked or broiled	3 oz	170
king, baked or broiled	3 oz	110
Mango, fresh, peeled, sliced	1 cup	110
Manicotti	2 pieces	300
Maple syrup		
regular	1 Tbsp	55
light/low calorie	1 Tbsp	20
Margarine		
regular	1 Tbsp	100
light/reduced fat (ranges from		

FOOD: (See Beverages & Fast Food Restaurants listed separately)	SERVING SIZE	CALORIES
20-70 calories/Tbsp, avg 45)	1 Tbsp	45
fat free	1 Tbsp	5
Marjoram, dried	1 tsp	2
Marmalade	1 Tbsp	50
Marshmallow		
4 large, or 1 oz	1 oz	90
Marshmallow topping	1 Tbsp	50
Mayonnaise		
regular	1 Tbsp	100
low calorie	1 Tbsp	25
Minestrone soup	1 cup	80
Molasses	1 Tbsp	55
Monkfish, meat only, broiled	3 oz	90
Mozzarella cheese – see cheese	…	…
Muenster cheese – see cheese	…	…
Muffin, 2 ½" dia		
apple, banana, or blueberry	1	165
bran	1	125
cinnamon raisin	1	145
chocolate	1	175
corn	1	160
English muffin, plain	1	130
raisin bran	1	185
Mulberries	½ cup	30
Mullet		
baked or broiled	3 oz	130
Mushrooms		
fresh, medium size	5	25
cut pieces, raw	½ cup	10
cut pieces, cooked	½ cup	20

FOOD: (See Beverages & Fast Food Restaurants listed separately)	SERVING SIZE	CALORIES
canned, slices, cooked	½ cup	25
Mussel blue, meat only, steamed	4 oz	195
Mustard regular hot or honey powder seeds	1 tsp 1 tsp 1 tsp 1 tsp	1 10 10 15
Mustard greens fresh, chopped, cooked frozen, cooked	½ cup ½ cup	10 15

FOOD: N through Z

FOOD: (See Beverages & Fast Food Restaurants listed separately)	SERVING SIZE	CALORIES
Nectarine, fresh, med, 2 ½" dia	1	65
Noodles plain, cooked fried, chow mein style	1 cup ½ cup	190 120
Nut pastry filling	1 Tbsp	65
Nuts, mixed, with peanuts dry roasted, about 20 nuts oil roasted, about 20 nuts	1 oz 1 oz	165 175
Oat bran	½ cup	225
Oat flour	½ cup	240
Oatmeal, as prep plain	¾ cup	100

FOOD: (See Beverages & Fast Food Restaurants listed separately)	SERVING SIZE	CALORIES
flavored oatmeal	¾ cup	150
Oats, dry, rolled,		
regular dry oats	½ cup	165
quick cooking dry oats	½ cup	150
Ocean Perch		
fresh, raw	3 oz	85
baked or broiled	3 oz	105
battered, fried	3 oz	180
Oil, vegetable		
for cooking, frying, and salads	1 Tbsp	120
non-stick cooking spray,		
¼ second spray	1 spray	0
Okra		
fresh or frozen, 3" pods	8 pods	30
fried, 3" pods	8 pods	115
sliced, cooked	½ cup	30
Olive		
green, stuffed or w/ pits		
1 svg = 4 small or 3 large	1 svg	15
ripe, mission, pitted		
1 svg = 3 med or 2 x-large	1 svg	15
Onion rings, 3" dia,		
battered, fried	2 rings	80
Onion soup broth	1 cup	45
Onion		
fresh, raw	2 oz	22
chopped, raw	2 Tbsp	5
chopped, cooked	½ cup	30
dried, flaked	1 Tbsp	15
green onion w/top, raw, chopped	½ cup	18

FOOD: (See Beverages & Fast Food Restaurants listed separately)	SERVING SIZE	CALORIES
Orange, fresh, medium size	1	60
Orange roughy, meat only, baked or broiled	3 oz	80

Oyster
  fresh, raw, meat only
  breaded, fried, large
  canned, drained
	4 oz
	3 oysters
	4 oz
		85
		155
		90

Pam, non-stick cooking spray ¼ second spray	1 spray	0

Pancake, plain
  prep from mix, 5" dia
  toaster size frozen pancakes
  toaster size lowfat pancakes
	1 piece
	1 piece
	1 piece
		90
		75
		50

Pancake syrup - see syrup	…	…
Papaya fresh, peeled, cubed	½ cup	25
Paprika	1 tsp	6
Parmesan cheese, grated	1 Tbsp	25

Parsley
  fresh, chopped
  dried
	¼ cup
	1 tsp
		6
		1

Parsnip, sliced, cooked	½ cup	65
Passion fruit, purple, trimmed	1 oz	25

Pasta
  plain, cooked
  prep w/tomato sauce and basil
	1 cup
	1 cup
		190
		215

Pasta sauce
  traditional tomato style sauce
  marinara
  with meat and mushrooms
	½ cup
	½ cup
	½ cup
		40
		75
		100

FOOD: (See Beverages & Fast Food Restaurants listed separately)	SERVING SIZE	CALORIES
Pastrami	2 oz	80
Pastry, Danish, 4" dia		
apple, cherry, any fruit variety	1 piece	385
cheese	1 piece	410
Pastry filling		
(also see individual listings)		
fruit flavored, avg calories	1 Tbsp	40
nut flavored, avg calories	1 Tbsp	65
Pea soup	1 cup	165
with ham added	1 cup	195
Peaches		
fresh, whole, medium size	1	40
fresh, sliced	½ cup	35
canned, in juice	½ cup	55
canned, in light syrup	½ cup	70
canned, in heavy syrup	½ cup	95
dried halves, unsweetened,		
cooked	½ cup	100
frozen, sliced, sweetened	½ cup	120
Peanut butter	2 Tbsp	190
Peanut, roasted, about 28 whole	1 oz	165
Pear		
fresh, med size	1	100
canned, in juice	½ cup	60
canned, in heavy syrup	½ cup	100
Peas		
black-eyed, cooked	½ cup	95
butter, cooked	½ cup	110
green or sweet, cooked	½ cup	65

FOOD: (See Beverages & Fast Food Restaurants listed separately)	SERVING SIZE	CALORIES
Peas and carrots equal mix, cooked	½ cup	55
Pecans, about 20 halves	1 oz	185
Pecan pastry filling	1 Tbsp	65

Pepper, dried powder
    black
    cayenne or red
    white
	
	1 tsp
	1 tsp
	1 tsp
		
		5
		7
		6

Pepperoni, 14 thin slices	1 oz	130

Peppers, fresh, sweet,
    red or green
        raw, whole, one med 3 ½" dia
        raw, chopped
        cooked, chopped
        yellow, one medium
	
	1
	½ cup
	½ cup
	1
		
		20
		17
		20
		30

Perch – see ocean perch	...	...
Pheasant, baked, meat only	4 oz	150

Pickle
    bread and butter chips, 4 pieces
    dill, 3 ¾" long
    sweet gherkin, 2 ½" long
	
	1 oz
	1
	1
		
		20
		5
		20

Pie,   1/8 of 9" pie
    apple, 2 crust pie
    blueberry, 2 crust pie
    cherry, 2 crust pie
    chocolate cream, 1 crust pie
    custard, 1 crust pie
    lemon meringue, 1 crust pie
    peach, 2 crust pie
    pecan, 1 crust pie
	
	1 slice
	1 slice
	1 slice
	1 slice
	1 slice
	1 slice
	1 slice
	1 slice
		
		455
		410
		405
		405
		285
		340
		405
		485

FOOD: (See Beverages & Fast Food Restaurants listed separately)	SERVING SIZE	CALORIES
pumpkin, 1 crust pie	1 slice	330
strawberry, 1 crust pie	1 slice	385
Pie crust		
9" regular crust	1 crust	750
9" graham crust	1 crust	850
Pierogie, cheese or onion	3	255
Pigs feet, pickled	2 oz	95
Pike, meat only, baked or broiled	3 oz	100
Pimiento	1 oz	10
Pineapple		
fresh, diced	½ cup	40
canned, chunks or tidbits		
in juice	½ cup	75
canned, chunks in heavy syrup	½ cup	100
canned, slices in juice	2 slices	55
canned, slices in heavy syrup	2 slices	75
Pistachio nuts, roasted, about 47	1 oz	170
Pizza		
(calories listed are for an		
avg slice, 1/8 of 9" pizza)		
cheese,		
thick pizza, thick crust	1 slice	200
thin pizza, thin crust	1 slice	120
hamburger or pepperoni,		
thick pizza, thick crust	1 slice	300
thin pizza, thin crust	1 slice	160
sausage or deluxe 2-3 meats,		
thick pizza, thick crust	1 slice	310
thin pizza, thin crust	1 slice	170

FOOD: (See Beverages & Fast Food Restaurants listed separately)	SERVING SIZE	CALORIES
Pizza rolls, 1 ½", frozen, as prep		
with cheese and one meat	5 pieces	170
with cheese and 2-3 meats	5 pieces	185
Pizza sauce	¼ cup	40
Plantain, sliced, cooked	½ cup	110
Plum		
fresh, med size	1	35
canned, in juice	½ cup	75
canned, in heavy syrup	½ cup	115
Polish sausage – see sausage	...	...
Pollock, meat only, baked or broiled	3 oz	100
Pomegranate, medium size, 9 oz	1	100
Pompano, baked or broiled	3 oz	175
Pop tarts toaster pastry, fruit, brown sugar, or chocolate		
frosted	1 pastry	200
plain	1 pastry	180
low fat	1 pastry	170
Popcorn		
air popped	1 cup	30
caramel coated	1 cup	75
cheese flavored	1 cup	50
microwave, butter flavored	1 cup	45
popped in vegetable oil	1 cup	45
reduced fat or light popcorn	1 cup	35
Poppyseed	1 tsp	15
Poppyseed pastry filling	1 Tbsp	70
Popsicle, fruit flavored	3 fl oz	70

FOOD: (See Beverages & Fast Food Restaurants listed separately)	SERVING SIZE	CALORIES
Pork (weights for meat only, w/o bones)		
Boston butt, roasted, lean	4 oz	275
lunch meat, thin sliced		
regular	2 slices	180
lowfat	2 slices	110
fat free	2 slices	60
picnic, shoulder, lean	3 oz	210
pork loin, roasted, lean and fat	4 oz	380
pork loin, roasted, lean only	4 oz	280
pork loin chop, lean and fat	4 oz	340
pork loin chop, lean only	4 oz	210
pork sausage, 1 patty or 2 links		
regular	2 oz	100
lowfat	2 oz	70
spare ribs, braised, lean with fat	3 oz	380
Pork rinds, deep fried, 1 cup	1 oz	150
Pot roast – see beef	...	...
Potato chips	10 chips	100
snack size pkg, 2 oz	1 pkg	300
barbecue, snack size pkg, 2 oz	1 pkg	320
Potatoes		
(see sweet potatoes listed separately)		
fresh, raw, whole as purchased	1 Lb	275
baked in skin, long type,		
1 medium, 4" x 2"	1 potato	150
boiled, peeled, round type,		
2 ½" dia	1 potato	110
boiled, peeled, diced or sliced	½ cup	60

FOOD: (See Beverages & Fast Food Restaurants listed separately)	SERVING SIZE	CALORIES
dehydrated flakes, mashed, as prep	½ cup	95
french fried, thin 3" strips	10	150
french fried, thick 3" strips	10	195
hash browned potatoes	½ cup	175
mashed, with milk and butter	½ cup	95
scalloped, au gratin with cheese	½ cup	155
Tater Tots type fried potatoes	10	150
Potpie, frozen, baked		
beef or pork, 8 oz pie	1 pie	490
chicken or turkey, 8 oz pie	1 pie	450
Pretzels		
Bavarian, twisted, 2 ½" x 3"	1	55
Dutch, twisted, 2 ½" x 3"	1	55
soft, twisted, 3" x 5"	1	180
sourdough, twisted, 2 ½" x 3"	1	55
sticks, 2 ½" long	10	20
snack size pkg, 2 oz	1 pkg	220
twists, 1 ½" dia	10	60
snack size pkg, 2 oz	1 pkg	220
Provolone cheese – see cheese	...	...
Prunes		
uncooked, unsweetened	5	85
dried, cooked, unsweetened	½ cup	100
dried, cooked, sweetened	½ cup	125
canned, in heavy syrup	½ cup	125
Pudding (regular is prep w/ whole milk) (lowfat & sugarfree are prep with 2% milk)		

FOOD: (See Beverages & Fast Food Restaurants listed separately)	SERVING SIZE	CALORIES
chocolate, regular	½ cup	160
lowfat	½ cup	100
sugarfree	½ cup	90
chocolate mousse, regular	½ cup	190
lowfat	½ cup	130
rice pudding, regular	½ cup	160
lowfat	½ cup	100
tapioca, regular	½ cup	130
lowfat	½ cup	90
sugarfree	½ cup	90
vanilla, regular	½ cup	140
lowfat	½ cup	90
sugarfree	½ cup	90
Pumpkin		
fresh, peeled and seeded	4 oz	30
canned	½ cup	40
Quesadillas, 1 average	1	500
Quiche Lorraine		
1/8 of 8" quiche	1 piece	470
Rabbit, meat only		
domesticated, stewed	4 oz	230
wild, stewed	4 oz	195
Radish, fresh, raw, med size	5	5
Raisin bran type cereal, 1 oz	½ cup	85
Raisins		
golden or natural	¼ cup	120
golden or natural 1.5 oz box	1 box	130
Ranch dip		
regular	1 Tbsp	30
fat free	1 Tbsp	15

FOOD: (See Beverages & Fast Food Restaurants listed separately)	SERVING SIZE	CALORIES
Raspberry		
fresh	½ cup	30
frozen, sweetened	½ cup	130
Ravioli, canned		
beef	1 cup	260
cheese	1 cup	225
Refried beans		
fat free	½ cup	110
regular	½ cup	130
w/black beans	½ cup	120
w/black beans and cheese	½ cup	135
w/sausage	½ cup	200
w/spicy hot sauce	½ cup	140
vegetarian	½ cup	110
Relish, sweet, finely chopped	1 Tbsp	20
Rhubarb		
fresh, diced	½ cup	14
cooked, sweetened	½ cup	140
Rice (as prepared)		
brown, plain	1 cup	200
long grain & wild, plain	1 cup	190
white, plain	1 cup	200
flavored- beef, chicken, pork	1 cup	270
fried rice- meatless	1 cup	280
fried rice- with meat or seafood	1 cup	310
herb & sauce rice dish	1 cup	240
pilaf rice dish	1 cup	250
spiced rice dish, Cajun	1 cup	240
vegetable rice dish	1 cup	240

FOOD: (See Beverages & Fast Food Restaurants listed separately)	SERVING SIZE	CALORIES
Rice cake		
regular size, all except sweet	1	35
regular size, sweetened	1	55
mini size, all except sweet	4	40
mini size, sweetened	4	60
Rice Chex cereal	1 cup	120
Rice Krispies cereal 1 oz	1 cup	110
Roast beef – see beef	…	…
Roast beef sandwich 2 ½ oz meat w/ sauce	1 avg	345
Rockfish, meat only, baked	3 oz	105
Rolls (also see bread)		
brown and serve roll, avg 0.8 oz	1	70
brown and serve, buttered	1	110
dinner roll, avg 1.0 oz	1	75
hard roll, avg 1.2 oz	1	85
kaiser, large, 2.2 oz	1	160
onion, large, 2.2 oz	1	160
poppy seed, large, 2.2 oz	1	170
sesame seed, large, 2.2 oz	1	170
sub roll, large, 2.2 oz	1	160
sweet roll, avg 1.6 oz	1	180
Rosemary, dried	1 tsp	4
Rutabaga, fresh, cooked, mashed	½ cup	45
Safflower seed kernels, dried	1 oz	145
Saffron	1 tsp	2
Sage, ground	1 tsp	2
Salad Dressing		
blue cheese, regular	1 Tbsp	75
blue cheese, low calorie	1 Tbsp	25

FOOD: (See Beverages & Fast Food Restaurants listed separately)	SERVING SIZE	CALORIES
buttermilk, regular	1 Tbsp	55
buttermilk, low calorie	1 Tbsp	15
Caesar, regular	1 Tbsp	55
Caesar, fat free	1 Tbsp	20
French, regular	1 Tbsp	60
French, low calorie	1 Tbsp	20
honey Dijon, regular	1 Tbsp	60
honey Dijon, fat free	1 Tbsp	25
Italian, regular	1 Tbsp	65
Italian, low calorie	1 Tbsp	15
mayonnaise, regular	1 Tbsp	100
mayonnaise, low calorie	1 Tbsp	25
olive oil, regular	1 Tbsp	35
ranch, regular	1 Tbsp	65
ranch, low calorie	1 Tbsp	20
Russian, regular	1 Tbsp	75
Russian, low calorie	1 Tbsp	25
thousand island, regular	1 Tbsp	65
thousand island, low calorie	1 Tbsp	20
Wish-Bone, regular	1 Tbsp	50
Wish-Bone, Lite	1 Tbsp	15
Salami	2 oz	140
Salisbury steak, *Dinty Moore*	1 svg	310
Salmon		
Atlantic, fresh, raw, meat only	3 oz	185
Chinook king salmon, raw, meat only	3 oz	190
red or pink salmon, baked or broiled	3 oz	155
red or pink salmon, smoked	3 oz	150

FOOD: (See Beverages & Fast Food Restaurants listed separately)	SERVING SIZE	CALORIES
silver coho salmon, canned in liquid, drained	3 oz	130
Salsa	1 Tbsp	6

Salt
  regular
  seasoned
	
	1 tsp
	1 tsp
		
		0
		5

Sandwich meat – see lunch meat	...	...

Sardines
  Atlantic, canned in oil, drained,
    7 medium
  Pacific, canned in mustard sauce
  Pacific, canned in tomato sauce
	
	3 oz
	3 oz
	3 oz
		
		175
		167
		168

Sauces
  (also see individual listings)
  A la king sauce
  Alfredo sauce, canned
  Alfredo sauce mix
  barbecue sauce, regular
    extra thick, or honey
  catsup
  cheese food spread
  cheese sauce
  chili sauce
  duck sauce, sweet & sour
  fish sauce, oriental
  hoison sauce
  hollandaise sauce
  horseradish sauce
  mustard
  oyster sauce
	
	½ cup
	½ cup
	1 pkg
	1 Tbsp
	1 Tbsp
	1 Tbsp
	1 Tbsp
	¼ cup
	¼ cup
	1 Tbsp
	1 Tbsp
	1 Tbsp
	1 Tbsp
	1 tsp
	1 tsp
	¼ cup
		
		40
		305
		180
		25
		40
		20
		45
		180
		60
		20
		7
		35
		10
		20
		5
		10

FOOD: (See Beverages & Fast Food Restaurants listed separately)	SERVING SIZE	CALORIES
sloppy Joe sauce	1 Tbsp	50
soy sauce	1 Tbsp	10
steak sauce	1 Tbsp	15
sweet & sour sauce	1 Tbsp	30
szechuan spice sauce	1 Tbsp	20
tartar sauce	1 Tbsp	45
teriyaki sauce	1 Tbsp	20
taco sauce	1 Tbsp	10
tomato sauce	½ cup	40
Sauerkraut, canned	½ cup	15
Sausage, 1 patty or 2 links		
regular beef or pork	2 oz	100
regular chicken or turkey	2 oz	85
lowfat variety	2 oz	70
Polish sausage, 5" x 2" link	1 link	250
Vienna sausage, canned, 2" long links	3 links	125
Scallop, meat only, baked	4 oz	105
Seaweed	1 sheet	10
Semolina, whole grain	½ cup	300
Sesame seeds	1 Tbsp	50
Shallot, chopped	1 Tbsp	7
Shark, meat only, battered, fried	4 oz	270
Sherbet, various flavors	½ cup	130
Shortening	1 Tbsp	120
Shredded wheat cereal		
spoon size, plain	1 cup	200
spoon size, frosted	1 cup	240
large biscuits, plain	3 pieces	220

FOOD: (See Beverages & Fast Food Restaurants listed separately)	SERVING SIZE	CALORIES
large biscuits, frosted	3 pieces	250
Shrimp		
canned	3 oz	95
fried	3 oz	195
steamed or boiled	3 oz	85
Sirloin steak – see beef	...	...
Smelt, rainbow, meat only, baked or broiled	3 oz	105
Snails (whelk), meat only, raw	4 oz	155
Snack mix, *Chex Mix*	1 cup	195
Snapper, meat only, broiled	3 oz	105
Sole, meat only		
baked or broiled	3 oz	90
breaded, fried	3 oz	170
Soup, as prep		
(Also see individual listings)		
bean and ham	1 cup	170
beef bouillon	1 cup	20
beef and vegetable	1 cup	120
broth, all types	1 cup	20
bouillon, all types	1 cube	20
clam chowder,		
Manhattan style	1 cup	80
New England style,		
prep with water	1 cup	95
prep with milk	1 cup	145
chicken broth	1 cup	20
chicken noodle soup	1 cup	75
chicken rice soup	1 cup	75
cream of broccoli soup	1 cup	235

FOOD: (See Beverages & Fast Food Restaurants listed separately)	SERVING SIZE	CALORIES
cream of chicken soup,		
prep with water	1 cup	115
prep with milk	1 cup	185
cream of mushroom soup,		
prep with water	1 cup	130
prep with milk	1 cup	190
onion soup w/mushrooms	1 cup	160
pea soup w/ham	1 cup	80
pea soup w/o meat	1 cup	140
tomato soup, prep with water	1 cup	85
vegetable soup, w/o meat	1 cup	70
vegetable soup, w/meat	1 cup	120
Sour cream		
regular	1 Tbsp	25
fat free	1 Tbsp	15
Soy sauce	1 Tbsp	10
Soybeans, dried mature seeds, cooked	½ cup	115
Spaghetti		
plain, cooked	1 cup	190
prep w/ tomato sauce	1 cup	210
prep w/ tomato & cheese sauce	1 cup	235
prep w/ meat balls in tomato sauce	1 cup	310
Spare Ribs – see pork	...	...
Special K cereal, 1 oz	1 ¼ cup	110
Spinach		
fresh, raw, chopped	1 cup	5
fresh or frozen, chopped, cooked	½ cup	22

FOOD: (See Beverages & Fast Food Restaurants listed separately)	SERVING SIZE	CALORIES
Squash, fresh		
acorn squash, baked, cubed	½ cup	55
summer, raw, sliced	½ cup	10
summer, sliced, cooked	½ cup	20
winter, baked, cubed	½ cup	40
winter, boiled, mashed	½ cup	45
Steak – see beef	...	...
Steak sauce	1 Tbsp	15
Strawberries		
fresh	½ cup	25
frozen, sweetened	½ cup	110
Stuffing, as prep		
traditional, seasoned	1 cup	120
chicken flavored	1 cup	150
corn bread stuffing	1 cup	125
Sturgeon, meat only		
baked or broiled	3 oz	120
smoked	3 oz	140
Sugar		
granulated (white) or brown	1 tsp	15
granulated (white) or brown	1 cup	720
powdered/confectioner's	1 tsp	10
powdered/confectioner's	1 cup	480
Sugar free gum & candy		
Sugar free gum, 2 7/8" stick	1 stick	5
Sugar free hard candy,		
Sweet'N Low, creme variety	1 piece	10
Sweet'N Low, misc varieties,		
except crème	1 piece	6

FOOD: (See Beverages & Fast Food Restaurants listed separately)	SERVING SIZE	CALORIES
Sugar substitute		
Equal or Sweet 'N Low	1 pkt	0
Sunflower seeds, roasted, hulled	2 Tbsp	105
Sweet potatoes		
fresh, raw, whole as purchased	1 Lb	410
baked or boiled in skin, 1 med	1 potato	170
boiled, peeled, mashed	½ cup	140
canned in liquid	½ cup	110
candied, 2 ½" x 2"	1 piece	145
Sweet 'N Low	1 pkt	0
Swordfish, meat only, baked	3 oz	130
Syrup		
butterscotch, regular	1 Tbsp	60
light/low calorie	1 Tbsp	25
chocolate, regular	1 Tbsp	60
light/low calorie	1 Tbsp	25
fruit flavored, regular	1 Tbsp	55
light/low calorie	1 Tbsp	20
pancake or maple syrup, regular	1 Tbsp	55
light/low calorie	1 Tbsp	20
Taco		
avg size, with meat	1	200
large, with meat	1	280
taco shell, thin, 6" dia	1	50
Tamale, canned	1 piece	90
Tangerine, fresh, med size	1	35
Tarragon, ground	1 tsp	5
Tarter sauce	1 Tbsp	45
Tater Tots type fried potatoes	10	150
T-bone steak – see beef	…	…

FOOD: (See Beverages & Fast Food Restaurants listed separately)	SERVING SIZE	CALORIES
Thyme, ground	1 tsp	4
Toaster pastry, fruit, brown sugar, or chocolate		
frosted, avg calories	1 pastry	200
plain, avg calories	1 pastry	180
low fat, avg calories	1 pastry	170
Tofu, plain, cooked, 4 oz	½ cup	80
Tomato		
fresh, raw, one med 2 ½" dia	1	25
fresh, boiled	½ cup	25
canned in liquid	½ cup	30
Tomato paste	¼ cup	60
Tomato sauce	½ cup	40
Tomato soup		
prep with water	1 cup	85
prep with milk	1 cup	145
Topping – see dessert topping and syrup	…	…
Total cereal, 1 oz	¾ cup	100
Trout, meat only, baked/broiled	3 oz	140
Tuna, light chunks		
canned in oil, drained	3 oz	170
canned in water, drained	3 oz	110
Tuna spread	2 Tbsp	50
Turkey lunch meat, thin sliced		
regular	2 slices	160
lowfat	2 slices	100
fat free	2 slices	50

FOOD: (See Beverages & Fast Food Restaurants listed separately)	SERVING SIZE	CALORIES
roasted turkey		
light meat, no skin	3 oz	135
light meat with skin	3 oz	165
dark meat, no skin	3 oz	160
dark meat with skin	3 oz	185
turkey liver, simmered	3 oz	180
Turkey sausage – see sausage	…	…
Turmeric, ground	1 tsp	8
Turnip greens, fresh or frozen Chopped, cooked	½ cup	18
Turnips, fresh		
raw, cubed	½ cup	20
cubed, cooked	½ cup	20
boiled, mashed	½ cup	25
Turnover fruit flavored, frozen, as prep		
small/mini *Pepperidge Farm*	1 piece	140
regular size *Pepperidge Farm*	1 piece	340
Vanilla extract	1 tsp	10
Veal cutlet, broiled	3 oz	185
Vegetable soup		
all vegetables, meatless	1 cup	70
with beef, chicken or turkey	1 cup	105

Vegetables
   (see individual listings)
   mixed vegetables, canned or
     frozen, w/o sauce, as prep
	½ cup	40

Venison, meat only, roasted	4 oz	175
Vienna Sausage – see sausage	…	…
Vinegar	1 Tbsp	0

FOOD: (See Beverages & Fast Food Restaurants listed separately)	SERVING SIZE	CALORIES
Waffle, toaster size	1 piece	100
Walnuts black, chopped (about ¼ cup) English (about 14 halves)	 1 oz 1 oz	 170 180
Water chestnut, canned, sliced	½ cup	75
Watermelon, fresh sliced wedge, 7" dia, 1" thick diced	 1 wedge ½ cup	 110 25
Wheat bran	¼ cup	25
Wheat germ	2 Tbsp	30
Wheaties cereal, 1 oz	1 cup	100
Whipped cream, pressurized	2 Tbsp	25
Whipped dessert topping frozen pressurized in can	 2 Tbsp 2 Tbsp	 30 25
Whiting, meat only, baked or broiled	 3 oz	 105
Wiener – see frankfurter	…	…
Wonton, Chinese, prep w/pork fried appetizer boiled, prep w/soup broth	 2 pieces 2 pieces	 125 70
Yam – see sweet potato	…	…
Yeast	¼ oz	20
Yogurt (average calories listed) plain, made w/ whole milk made w/ lowfat milk made w/ skim milk fruit or flavored varieties, made w/ whole milk made w/ lowfat milk	 8 oz 8 oz 8 oz 8 oz 8 oz	 140 130 125 250 210

FOOD: (See Beverages & Fast Food Restaurants listed separately)	SERVING SIZE	CALORIES
made w/ skim milk	8 oz	175
Zucchini		
fresh, 1 medium size	1	5
boiled, sliced	½ cup	15
canned, in tomato sauce	½ cup	30

EZ LIFETIME
A TO Z
CALORIE COUNTER©

FAST FOOD RESTAURANTS

FAST FOOD RESTAURANT: (See other Foods and Beverages listed separately)	SERVING SIZE	CALORIES
Arby's		
Arby's sauce	1 pkt	15
Beef & cheddar	1	450
Biscuit w/bacon	1	360
Club sandwich	1	560
Coleslaw	1 svg	85
Croissant w/bacon	1	340
French fries	1 svg	300
Ham & cheese	1	380
Jr. Roast beef	1	220
Roast Beef	1	350
Shake, chocolate or vanilla	14 oz	490
Turkey sandwich	1	410
Turkey deluxe sandwich	1	510
Burger King		
Apple pie	1	240
Biscuit w/bacon, egg, and cheese	1	620
BK Broiler chicken sandwich	1	530
Cheeseburger	1	350
Cini-mini's (without icing)	4	440

FAST FOOD RESTAURANT: (See other Foods and Beverages listed separately)	SERVING SIZE	CALORIES
Chicken tenders	8	350
Croissan'wich w/sausage, egg, and cheese	1	530
Double beef whopper	1	850
Hamburger	1	290
French fries, medium	1 svg	375
Onion rings, medium	1 svg	380
Shake, vanilla or chocolate	1	430
Whopper	1	630
Whopper Jr.	1	400
Whopper w/ cheese	1	730
Domino's Pizza		
Breadstick	1	80
Cheesy bread, large slice	1 slice	100
Deep Dish Pizza, cheese, 6", whole	1 pizza	595
Hand-tossed cheese pizza	2 lg slices	315
Hand-tossed mushroom pizza	2 lg slices	320
Hand-tossed pepperoni pizza	2 lg slices	370
Dunkin' Donuts		
Bagels & cream cheese		
plain or onion	1	335
poppyseed or sesame	1	370
all other bagels	1	350
Cream cheese,		
light	1 pkt	130
regular or flavored	1 pkt	190
Bow tie donut	1	300
Cake donut, regular size		
frosted	1	230

FAST FOOD RESTAURANT: (See other Foods and Beverages listed separately)	SERVING SIZE	CALORIES
fruit flavored or chocolate	1	295
glazed	1	270
powdered	1	250
Cinnamon bun	1	510
Cookie, avg calories	1	225
Cruller, glazed	1	290
Jelly filled donut	1	210
"Kreme" filled donut, avg	1	270
Muffin, 4 oz, all except lowfat	1	350
Muffin, lowfat	1	245
Munchkins, cake type, avg	3	200
Munchkins, yeast type, avg	3	210
Yeast donut, regular size		
frosted	1	270
fruit flavored or chocolate	1	280
glazed	1	210
"Kreme" filled type	1	270
Hardees		
All-star burger	1	660
Biscuit 'n gravy	1	530
Chicken biscuit	1	590
Cole slaw	1 svg	240
Crispy curls potatoes, large	1 svg	520
Famous star burger	1	570
Fisherman's fillet sandwich	1	530
French fries, small	1 svg	240
Frisco burger	1	720
Grilled chicken sandwich	1	350
Hamburger	1	270
Jelly biscuit	1	440

FAST FOOD RESTAURANT: (See other Foods and Beverages listed separately)	SERVING SIZE	CALORIES
Regular roast beef	1	310
Sausage biscuit	1	550
Shake, 12 oz	1	400
Super star	1	790
Twist cone	1	180
Kentucky Fried Chicken		
BBQ baked beans	1 svg	190
Biscuit	1	180
Chicken sandwich	1	495
Value BBQ chicken sandwich	1	255
Cole slaw	1 svg	180
Cornbread	1	225
Extra crispy fried chicken		
breast	1	470
drumstick	1	190
thigh	1	370
wing	1	200
Mashed potatoes w/gravy	1 svg	120
Original recipe fried chicken		
breast	1	400
drumstick	1	140
thigh	1	250
wing	1	140
Potato salad	1 svg	230
Potato wedges	1 svg	280
Tender roast, without skin		
breast	1	170
drumstick	1	70
thigh	1	105

FAST FOOD RESTAURANT: (See other Foods and Beverages listed separately)	SERVING SIZE	CALORIES
Long John Silvers		
Calories listed are for "Dinners", including hushpuppies & fries		
2 piece Chicken Dinner	1	990
2 piece Fish Dinner	1	970
3 piece Chicken Dinner	1	1190
3 piece Fish Dinner	1	1160
McDonald's		
Apple pie	1	260
Big mac	1	560
Cheeseburger	1	320
Chicken mcnuggets	6 pieces	290
Egg mcmuffin	1	290
Filet-o-fish sandwich	1	430
French fries, small	1 svg	220
French fries, large	1 svg	450
Garden salad, without dressing	1	35
Grilled chicken deluxe, without mayonnaise	1	300
Hamburger	1	260
Hash browns	1 patty	130
Honey	1 pkg	45
Honey or hot mustard	1 pkg	55
Light mayonnaise	1 pkg	40
McDonaldland cookies	1 pkg	180
Muffin, banana, blueberry, orange, or chocolate chip	1	415
Quarter pounder	1	430
Quarter pounder w/cheese	1	530

FAST FOOD RESTAURANT: (See other Foods and Beverages listed separately)	SERVING SIZE	CALORIES
Sausage biscuit w/egg	1	550
Shake, chocolate, vanilla, or strawberry	1 small	360
Salad dressing, ranch	1 pkg	230
Fat free herb vinaigrette	1 pkg	50
Reduced calorie French	1 pkg	160
Pizza Hut		
Bread stick	1	130
Cheese pizza, thin 'n crispy	1 slice	240
Meat lover's pizza	1 slice	380
Pepperoni, thin 'n crispy	1 slice	240
Personal pan pizza, pepperoni	1 pizza	620
Stuffed crust, cheese	1 slice	360
Stuffed crust, meat lover's	1 slice	470
Thin 'n crispy pizza with cheese and 1 meat	1 slice	250
Thick or Pan pizza w/cheese and 1 meat	1 slice	350
Veggie lover's pizza	1 slice	280
Subway		
6 Inch cold sub		
Italian BMT	1	450
Veggie delight	1	230
Other cold subs, avg calories	1	300
6 Inch hot sub		
Meatball	1	415
Other hot subs, avg calories	1	350
Deli style sandwich	1	240
Fruizle smoothie	12 oz	130

FAST FOOD RESTAURANT: (See other Foods and Beverages listed separately)	SERVING SIZE	CALORIES
Super subs		
Italian BMT	1	670
Cold cut trio	1	515
Subway club	1	370
Wraps, meat and cheese, 9 oz	1	350
Taco Bell		
7-Layer burrito, 10 oz	1	530
Bean burrito	1	380
Burrito supreme	1	440
Cinnamon twists	1 svg	140
Chicken fajita wrap	1	460
Chicken fajita wrap supreme	1	520
Grilled chicken burrito	1	400
Mexican rice	1 svg	190
Nachos	1 svg	320
Pintos 'n cheese	1 svg	190
Santa Fe beef gordita	1	380
Soft taco	1	220
Soft taco supreme	1	260
Taco	1	180
Taco supreme	1	220
Taco salad w/salsa, w/ shell	1	850
Taco salad w/salsa, no shell	1	420
Tostada	1	300
Wendy's		
Baked potato, plain	1	310
Baked potato, bacon & cheese	1	530
Baked potato, broccoli,cheese	1	470
Baked potato, w/sour cream	1	380
Chicken sandwich, breaded	1	440

FAST FOOD RESTAURANT: (See other Foods and Beverages listed separately)	SERVING SIZE	CALORIES
Chicken sandwich, grilled	1	310
Chili, small	1 svg	210
French fries, medium	1 svg	420
Frosty dairy dessert, small	1	330
Grilled chicken salad w/ light dressing	1	240
Hamburger, plain	1	360
Hamburger w/everything	1	420
Pita, chicken Caesar	1	490
Pita, classic Greek	1	440
Pita, garden ranch chicken	1	480
Pita, garden veggie	1	400
Taco salad w/light dressing	1	420

NOTES

EZ! LIFETIME DIET & EXERCISE GUIDE

By: Helena Schaar

You can be in total control of your weight forever. The facts, tips, and ideas in this guide give you the "need to know" essentials of calories, exercise, and weight management. This guide along with the calorie counter gives you the power and the knowledge to control your weight forever.

These lifetime weight management ideas promote good health. This plan is safe, effective, easy to follow, and fits into any lifestyle. Learn the secrets to weight management, and simple exercise routines that lead to a lifetime of health, well being, and total success in weight control.

Fad diets, crash diets, and starvation diets are not recommended. You may lose weight, however, as soon as you resume your normal eating habits, the weight will return. There are also potential adverse health effects from any type of quick weight loss diet. Starvation diets also lead to a slower metabolism.

For total lifetime control of your weight, it is better to have a diet plan you can easily live with forever; one that does not feel like a diet at all!

Please Note: As with any weight management plan, results may vary for each individual. You should always consult your physician before beginning any new diet or exercise plan; and especially if you have current health problems, or you are pregnant or nursing. This diet plan is offered only as information, for use in maintaining and promoting your good health in cooperation with a physician. In the event that the information presented in this diet plan is used without a physician's approval, the individual using the plan accepts all responsibility. This plan is only intended for normal healthy adults over age 20. Those with underlying health problems may or may not be able to achieve their weight goals, or maintain their weight goals. Always consult your physician first.

This diet plan is very simple: You first choose your ideal body weight. You may know exactly what is right for you, or you can refer to the "Ideal Body Weight" chart. You then calculate the number of daily calories needed to achieve that weight. (Calculations discussed later). You can eat satisfying and well-balanced variety of foods, including all your favorite foods, while making better food choices by counting calories. Read over the Healthy Diet Basics, and the EZ Weight Loss Secrets. If you want to achieve optimal health, you should add a simple exercise routine to your day. Exercise also helps speed up weight loss, and makes lifetime weight management much easier.

When trying to lose weight, several factors come into play that affect the speed of weight loss. This includes:

- How many pounds you are above your ideal weight. Generally, the more you weigh, the faster you will lose weight. Losing 5 to 7 pounds per month is a healthy goal if you are overweight.
- Your commitment to counting and cutting calories and your commitment to get active with exercise.
- Your metabolism. As you age, metabolism naturally slows down. Exercise speeds up the metabolism. Heredity is also a factor; some naturally have a faster metabolism than others.

HEALTHY DIET BASICS

The following is a list of important facts, and healthy tips to keep in mind for smart weight management. These tips will help in achieving and maintaining your ideal weight.

Drink 6 to 8 glasses of water every day. Water helps to cleanse and purify the body, and improves overall health.

Take a multi-vitamin and mineral supplement every day. This helps to assure that you are obtaining all the essential nutrients your body needs.

Eat a variety of foods every day from all of the food groups. Variety and balance in the food groups helps to assure proper nutrition and good health. All types of foods contain varying amounts of vitamins, minerals, and nutrients. The food groups are:

- Bread, grains, oats, wheat, cereal, rice, and pasta. (Good source of carbs and fiber, some protein).

- Fruits and vegetables. (Fruits high in carbs; vegetables contain many nutrients, plus some protein and fiber).

- Dairy products including milk, and cheese. (High in protein and carbs, some are high in fat).

- Meat products including beef, pork, chicken, fish, and eggs. (High in protein, some are high in fat).

- Fats, oils, and sweets. Minimize intake of this food group. (Very high in fat and/or sugar).

The USDA recommendations for variety and balance in daily caloric intake follows:

- 50% to 60% from carbohydrates (carbs)
- 12% to 20% from proteins
- Less than 30% from fats

For example, in an 1800 calorie diet, for a 120 pound adult, the USDA recommends the following daily intake for optimal nutritional health:

Carbohydrates: 250 grams
             (about 55% of total caloric intake)

Protein: 54 grams
             (about 16% of total caloric intake,
               or 0.45 grams/kg of body weight)

Fat: Less than 58 grams
             (less than 30% of total caloric intake)

Fiber: 23 grams or more. Fiber is good for you with multiple health benefits. Fiber is especially good for the heart and colon. Some studies indicate that an increase in fiber with the proper balance of protein increases the metabolism naturally, resulting in faster weight loss, and easier weight management.

Carbohydrates can be classified as simple, such as sugar, or complex. The complex carbs are good for you and contain many nutrients. Carbohydrates also include fiber, which is very good for you. Foods high in complex carbs, such as bread and rice contain many vitamins and minerals. Carbs also contain starch and sugar. Sugar is the so-called "bad carb", high in calories with little nutritional value. You can usually tell a bad carb because it is sweet.

Increased focus has been given to diets that promote very high intake of protein, with very low intake of carbohydrates. This does promote fast weight loss in many people. However, nutrition experts agree that a well balanced diet with higher intake of carbohydrates, less protein, and less fat is safer and healthier. A minor increase in protein intake, with a minor decrease in carbohydrate intake is a better option if considering a high protein diet. The extremes of almost all protein and fat, with almost no carbohydrate intake can have serious health consequences. Health problems noted in high protein, high fat, low carb diets include: kidney failure, increased risk of heart disease due to increased cholesterol levels, and increased risk of cancer.

ALL ABOUT CALORIES & WEIGHT

Simply put, if you eat fewer calories, you will lose weight. There are 3500 calories in one pound. For every 3500 calories you cut out of your diet, you will lose one pound of body weight. Calories provide energy. You need calories and the energy derived from calories to live. However, if you consume more calories than your body needs, the result is weight gain. For the safest, healthiest weight loss, you need to maintain the proper caloric intake, balance your food groups, and increase your physical activity level. This leads to good health, good nutrition, and easy to maintain, long lasting results.

You can choose your perfect weight for yourself, or refer to the ideal body weight chart. Then you just determine the number of calories you need per day to achieve that weight. For example: Let's say your ideal perfect weight is 120 pounds, and you have a moderately active lifestyle. You need 1800 calories per day. (See the lifestyle activity levels and factors). No matter what your present weight is, if you begin today to eat 1800 calories per day, and you are a moderately active healthy adult, you will eventually weigh 120 pounds. It's that easy. 1800 calories per day is a satisfying amount of food, it certainly does not seem like a diet to most people. 1800 calories per day leaves plenty of room for good variety, balance, and nutrition. You just need to learn to make smart food choices, and counting calories is the best way.

Read over the calorie counter. Get to know which foods are naturally lower in calories. Reducing your caloric intake, and managing your weight is so much easier once you learn which types of foods are high in calories, and which types of foods are low in calories.

Do you need to spend lots of time counting every calorie?

No. Calorie counting gets easier over time, and after a while it is like second nature. After a few months of using a calorie counter, most people have memorized the approximate calorie counts of favorite foods. While it is true every calorie counts in weight management, it is also true that every bit of activity also counts. It is almost impossible to measure exactly how many calories you burn in a day; you would have to measure calorie expenditure every time you stand up, even every time you move. It is, however, easy to figure approximately how many calories you need, and how many you burn per day with the simple formulas in this book. So, you do not need to spend lots of time counting every calorie. Instead, try rounding and averaging calories to save time, but don't cheat yourself by neglecting to count the majority of your calories.

An easy calorie counting tip is to start the day with 200 calories as a catch-all for any tiny snacks like sugar free candy or gum, diet sodas, other diet beverages, celery or carrot sticks, etc. Then, say for an example, your ideal weight is 120 pounds, and you are a moderately active person. You get to consume 1800 calories per day. Subtract the 200 calorie catch-all, and you have about 1600 calories to divide over 3 meals. After some practice counting calories, you won't even need to write down the daily calorie counts, you will be easily able to keep a daily running total in the back of your mind.

How many calories do you need per day?

There are complicated formulas and expensive tests to determine your caloric requirements based on basal metabolism. A very simple rule of thumb is to choose your ideal weight (the weight you consider perfect for yourself) and multiply by 15 to determine your daily caloric requirements. This formula is correct for moderately active, healthy adults over age 20. The activity levels and factors are discussed in the next section.

If you are extremely active, your caloric requirements will be higher. If you are sedentary, your caloric requirements will be lower.

(Notes: Caloric requirements decrease with age as the metabolism slows down. Caloric requirements can be significantly increased during any illness.)

FORMULA FOR CALCULATING DAILY CALORIES NEEDED:

Multiply your ideal body weight by your activity factor to determine daily caloric requirements.

Example: A moderately active adult who wants to weigh 120 pounds, needs 1800 calories per day.

$$120 \times 15 = 1800$$

CALORIE EXPENDITURE & EXERCISE

Calorie expenditure describes the process of the body utilizing or burning calories for energy. Different activities burn calories at different levels. You can measure your overall lifestyle activity level and the factors by using this chart. You can then make adjustments to your activity level, and add exercises that help burn calories faster.

LIFESTYLE ACTIVITY LEVELS & FACTORS

Sedentary Lifestyle   (Factor = 12)
  Sitting most of the day, no formal exercise program.

Moderately Active Lifestyle   (Factor = 15)
  Performs regular moderately strenuous exercise program at least 3 times per week for at least 20 minutes per session. Good amount of walking and activity in normal daily routine.

Vigorously Active Lifestyle   (Factor = 18)
  Extremely active. Performs regular strenuous exercise at least 5 times per week for at least 30 minutes per session. Exercise program includes running or jogging at fast pace, high impact aerobic type exercise, or equally strenuous exercise. Daily routine and/or job include lots of physical activity.

If you fall somewhere in the middle, your activity factor will fall somewhere in the middle of these activity factors.

Tip: Every time you perform a physical activity or exercise, you are burning more calories than if you are sitting. So a key to losing weight faster, is to GET ACTIVE! Take the stairs whenever possible, take a walk after eating, find an exercise or activity you enjoy, and add it to your daily routine. Adding a simple exercise like walking, biking, or swimming to your daily routine, for 20 minutes per day, 3 to 5 days per week will help to speed up weight loss, increase muscle tone, and increase your energy level.

Which exercises burn more calories?

Simply, the more strenuous the exercise, the more calories you burn. You can also gauge how vigorous the exercise is by checking your heart rate.

Weight training/weightlifting is a little different than other exercises. You may or may not increase you heart rate as much as with other exercises, but you are still doing yourself a world of good. Weight training is very effective at toning muscles and increasing lean muscle mass. This means you will have less fat and more muscle on your body. Muscle also weighs more than fat, so you will need more calories per day to maintain your weight. You can also achieve your ideal physique by adjusting the amount of weights you train with, and the number of repetitions you perform. You can choose to be anywhere from slim and well toned to very muscular. Most women prefer the slim and well-toned look. To achieve that, use light weights and more repetitions. Two to five pound weights that can be held in each hand are ideal. Lift them over your head in slow repetitions for 10 minutes, and work your way up to 20 minutes. Perform this exercise 3 times per week. This can be combined with riding an indoor stationary bike to save time, and get an all over workout.

An exercise is classified as aerobic if you can achieve and maintain your maximum heart rate range for at least 20 minutes, and preferably 30 minutes. Aerobic exercise provides a multitude of health benefits. This includes:

- Increased energy levels
- Faster weight loss
- Improved overall health
- Lower blood pressure and lower resting heart rate (This is a long-term beneficial aspect of aerobic exercise).

Before beginning an exercise, check your normal resting heart rate. The normal for an adult is 60 to 100 beats per minute, with 80 being the average normal value. Count the heartbeat for 15 seconds and multiply by 4 to calculate beats per minute. Then check your heart rate periodically while performing an exercise, to be sure you are maintaining the aerobic level.

Using heart rate to calculate aerobic exercise level:

Your target heart rate while exercising is calculated as follows:

220 (minus your age) x (75% to 85%)

Example: for a 35 year old female:
220 – 35 = 185 x 75% = 139

In this example, the 35 year old female can gauge the exercise activity level by her heart rate increase from a resting heart rate of 80 to the aerobic exercise heart rate of 139. The heart rate should be checked periodically to gauge the aerobic level.

Note: If your heart rate is much higher than calculated in the formula, you should stop exercising, and consult your physician before restarting aerobic exercise. Using 85% in the formula above instead of 75% is the maximum heart rate you should achieve. Also, any illness including a fever can increase heart rate, so the heart rates given here are for normal healthy adults only. Always check with your doctor before beginning any exercise program.

Calorie expenditure chart*

Calorie expenditure increases with more strenuous exercise and activity. This chart reveals some common activities and the number of calories burned per hour during these activities.

*Calories burned per hour in this example are approximate values for a normal healthy adult female weighing 130 pounds, or a normal, healthy adult male weighing 165 pounds.

Activity/Exercise	*Calories burned per hour	
	Female	Male
Sitting quietly	60	80
Standing still	75	100

Light activity/exercise
  Cleaning the house
  Walking slowly/strolling
  Playing golf
	210	250

Moderate activity/exercise
  Bicycling at 6 mph
  Fast power walking at 3.5 mph
  Swimming at a moderate pace
  Low/Moderate impact aerobics
  Dancing at moderate pace
  Moderate weight training
  Playing basketball
  Playing tennis
	330	410

Strenuous activity/exercise	620	800

  High impact aerobics
  Swimming very fast
  Jogging/running at 8 mph or faster
  Jumping rope very fast
  Stair stepping
  Cross country skiing

ACTIVITY/EXERCISE TIPS:

Choose an activity you enjoy, and perform it regularly for 20 minutes per day at least three days per week. This will promote faster weight loss, easier weight management, improved overall health, and improved sense of well being.

This exercise can be as simple as walking. You can walk outside and get the added benefit of fresh air, or if the weather is poor, you can simulate a walk inside while watching your favorite television program, or catching up on the news. You should walk at a fast pace, but one that is comfortable to you. Don't walk so fast that you get short of breath. Your stamina and endurance will increase the longer you continue. If you are walking inside, be sure to really lift your feet off the floor. Whether indoors or outdoors, you should swing your arms back and forth, or continuously lift them over your head as if reaching for the sky. This provides for all-over muscle toning. If you want to tone up your arm muscles faster, and burn lots of extra calories, you can hold weights in your hands while you walk. Another option is to strap weights to your ankles. Two or three pound weights are ideal, very easy to find, and very inexpensive.

Bicycling is also a very enjoyable exercise for many. This can be done indoors on a stationary bike or outdoors in the fresh air. Indoor bikes should have tension controls so you can adjust your calorie expenditure based on endurance. Here again, weights can be used to burn lots of extra calories and tone the arms. Two or three pound weights are ideal. Hold them in your hands and lift upward in repetitions. If biking outdoors, find routes with hills, if possible, for maximum calorie expenditure.

Once you have mastered one exercise, you can step up to a higher activity level exercise. Read over the list to see which ones burn more calories, and find one you truly enjoy. Once you have achieved your ideal weight, continue the exercise routine, or even step up a level, to maintain your optimal good health and your ideal weight.

EZ! Weight Loss Secrets

Try one, two, or all of these tips for easy weight loss. Step on the scale a week later, or a month later and be amazed at the results! Be sure to also follow the Healthy Diet Basics outlined earlier.

- Many of your favorite foods come in low calorie, light, sugar free, low fat, and fat free versions that are almost equal in taste. Try it, you might like it!

- By switching to the sugar free or calorie-free version of most of your beverages, you can cut your daily caloric intake considerably; even up to 800 calories per day, with very little effort. The result of switching to the low calorie versions of foods and drinks is fast and easy weight loss. Try it for ¼, or ½, or more of the foods and beverages you consume, and be amazed at the results. Of course, it is impractical to do this for all of your foods. Everyone wants to enjoy special foods and drinks for holidays, special occasions, eating out with friends, and just because it's good to treat yourself. After the special occasions, you can easily get right back into the pattern of healthy eating.

- When you choose foods in the low calorie, light, sugar free, low fat, or fat free versions, you save anywhere from 10% to 90% of the calories for that dish. For example, a rice dish made with 1 tablespoon of regular butter has 250 calories. If you use fat free margarine instead of regular butter, the total calories are about 150, saving you 100 calories. A salad with 2 tablespoons of fat free dressing instead of regular dressing saves you about 120 calories.

- Prepare your food without adding cooking oil that has 120 calories per tablespoon. Try baking, broiling, or grilling with a non-stick cooking spray that has zero calories.

- With sugar free fruit flavored beverages like *Crystal Light* or *Kool Aid*, you can save about 100 calories per cup over regular fruit flavored beverages. These come in many varieties and are excellent thirst quenchers. With soft drinks, you can reduce the calories from about 150 to zero by switching to a diet version of the soda.

- For between meal snacks, try anything low calorie, and low fat. Some examples are sugar free gum and candy, vegetables with fat free dip, carrot sticks, and any diet beverage. With just a small snack you will easily be able to curb your cravings for an hour or two until your next meal.

- Choose foods that are low in fat, salt, and sugar, these foods are naturally lower in calories and promote weight loss.

- Add a little physical activity at least three to five days per week. Read the "All About Calories" topic which includes calorie expenditure charts as related to exercise. To begin, choose a simple and pleasant exercise such as walking, swimming, or riding a bicycle. Just 20 minutes per day, a few days per week, can dramatically accelerate your weight loss, increase energy levels, and improve your overall sense of well being. Your brain releases endorphins when you exercise. Endorphins are chemicals that make you feel good, and the feeling can last for many hours after you finish exercising. Many people who exercise regularly say they feel energized all day long. Let the endorphins flow!

****

Good luck and the best of health to you, and happy calorie counting!

****

Ideal Body Weight Chart

The following chart is to help you calculate your ideal body weight. This chart is for adults age 20 and over. The data is compiled from various medical and health journals. There is a wide range of what is considered to be the "ideal" body weight. This chart lists weights for a medium frame, with one to two pounds of clothing on. Heights listed are without shoes. You should only weigh yourself in the morning, before eating or drinking anything. This is the best way to track the trend of your weight loss, since your weight can fluctuate throughout the day, especially after eating a meal. You should use this chart only as an estimated guide to your ideal weight.

FEMALE:

Height (Feet' Inches")	Ideal Body Weight (in Pounds)
5'0"	100 – 110
5'1"	102 – 112
5'2"	105 – 118
5'3"	108 – 122
5'4"	110 – 125
5"5"	114 – 130
5'6"	116 – 136
5'7"	120 – 140
5'8"	125 – 145
5'10"	130 – 155

MALE:

Height (Feet'Inches")	Ideal Body Weight (in Pounds)
5'4"	125 – 140
5'6"	135 – 155
5'8"	145 – 165
5'10"	160 – 175
6'0"	170 – 185
6'2"	180 – 195

****

Free Access to Internet Site with Complete Food Nutritional Values

This website is the USDA database of complete nutritional food counts. This database includes gram and milligram counts for carbohydrates (carbs), protein, fat, fiber, sodium, cholesterol, calcium, and much, much more.

The USDA also provides a wealth of health and diet information completely free to the public! There you can find the food guide pyramid, and the Recommended Daily Intake values of essential nutrients.

The data is in an easy to download, save, and print file that is approximately 105 pages long. Finding all of this information in one printable PDF file is quite a task with the ever-expanding world wide web, but this is the ultimate nutritional site. The website address is:

www.nal.usda.gov/fnic/foodcomp/Data/HG72/ hg72.html

You then click on HG-72, and you have your complete nutrition book. If you ever have trouble accessing the site, simply go to usda.gov, and search for the "Home and Garden Bulletin". The bulletin is edition 72, completely updated and revised in 2002.

****

CALORIE & EXERCISE NOTES

DATE	CALORIES CONSUMED	EXERCISE TYPE & TIME	WEIGHT

CALORIE & EXERCISE NOTES

DATE	CALORIES CONSUMED	EXERCISE TYPE & TIME	WEIGHT

NOTES

About the author:

Helena Schaar is a licensed, registered, healthcare professional with over 15 years of experience. Helena works as a healthcare therapist, educator, and medical writer with over 30 published articles. These articles have been recognized, approved, and accredited by state and national healthcare licensing boards.

Helena and her family live in the sunshine state of Florida. Helena is a lifelong devotee of health and fitness, including calorie counting, good nutrition and plenty of exercise.

Printed in the United States
89106LV00008B/23/A

9 781411 602823